OLDER,
WISER,
FIERCER!

VIRGINIA WILDE

♀LDER,
WISER,
FIERCER!

The Wit and
Wisdom of Women

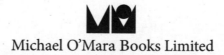

Michael O'Mara Books Limited

First published in Great Britain in 2023 by
Michael O'Mara Books Limited
9 Lion Yard
Tremadoc Road
London SW4 7NQ

A CIP catalogue record for this book is available from the British Library.

Papers used by Michael O'Mara Books Limited are natural, recyclable products
made from wood grown in sustainable forests. The manufacturing processes
conform to the environmental regulations of the country of origin.

ISBN: 978-1-78929-576-4 in hardback print format
ISBN: 978-1-78929-577-1 in ebook format

1 2 3 4 5 6 7 8 9 10

Cover design by Ana Bjezancevic
Internal illustrations by Jenny Wren
Pattern assets from shutterstock.com
Designed and typeset by Jade Wheaton
Printed and bound by CPI Group (UK) Ltd, Croydon, CR0 4YY

www.mombooks.com

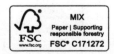

For all the fierce and fabulous women out there.

May we get fiercer and even more fabulous with each passing year.

Contents

Introduction

Older, Wiser, Fiercer

The joy and freedom that comes with being an older woman is probably one of life's best-kept secrets.

Sure, there are downsides (a number of things are in fact further down from where they once were). But though we may no longer have the ability to stay up late with no consequences or sit down without making a quiet 'oof' noise, if this is the price of self-knowledge and not really caring what anyone else thinks then that is a pretty good deal.

In the past, older women were called witches and feared for practising dark magic. Which makes absolute sense because we do have special powers and they should be scared.

No one gets this far down the road of life – navigating all of its potholes, diversions, dead ends and idiotic other drivers – without learning a thing or two. When you have dealt with enough recalcitrant toddlers, stroppy teenagers and difficult bosses (oddly similar); when you have chosen partners, sofas and wedding guest outfits; when you have lived through family crises, plumbing emergencies and realizing the price sticker is still on the sole of your shoe, nothing really fazes you anymore.

We also had the distinct advantage of growing up in the pre-social-media age. Young people today have their every moment photographed and filmed in high definition and uploaded to the internet. Thank goodness no one was recording the things we got up to in *our* youth . . .

It's true that older women are sometimes overlooked and patronized. It can feel like we have as much chance of attracting the attention of a young sales assistant in a phone shop as we do of winning the lottery. But even this can be an advantage, because what it means is that *no one suspects an older woman.*

'The trick is to age honestly and gracefully and make it look great, so that everyone looks forward to it.'

Emma Thompson

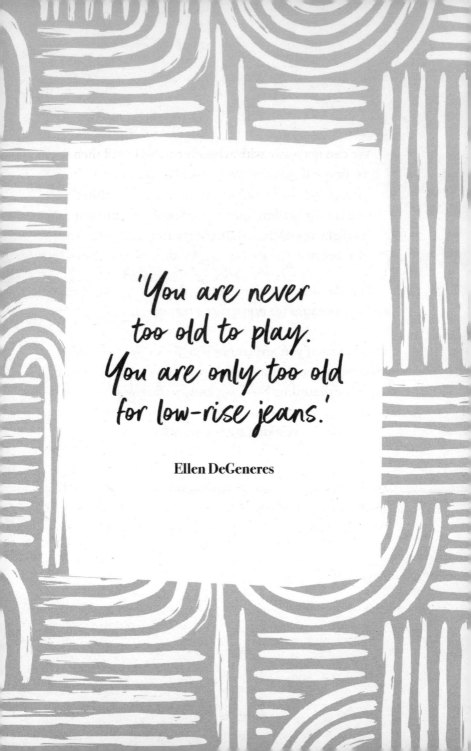

'You are never
too old to play.
You are only too old
for low-rise jeans.'

Ellen DeGeneres

We can get away with whatever we like and then fake-limp off into the sunset like Keyser Soze at the end of *The Usual Suspects*. If young people think that we are settling quietly and boringly into our 'twilight years' then that's fine with us. We don't care because we are having the time of our lives.

And the reason we are having the time of our lives is precisely because we don't care anymore. Or at least, we are very selective about what we choose to give a rat's ass about. When you are young you are so worried about what other people think and what you should be doing that it is exhausting. So if we look tired now, it's because being young was draining – being older is so much more relaxing by comparison.

So let's raise a glass to the wisdom and joy that comes with older age. To our wrinkles and our random chin hairs and to knowing who we are and what we like. We are funny, we are fierce and yes, we might just be witches too.

Socializing

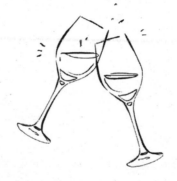

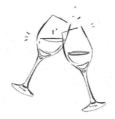

In our twenties, we dashed around, hating to refuse an invitation, scared of missing something exciting. Now it's more a case of figuring out how to charmingly get out of most of the invites we do get.

It's not that we want to become grumpy old hermits, used to our own strange habits while totally intolerant of the eccentricities of others. It's simply that we know who we like and what we enjoy. If a party is dull, we leave it. If a trip sounds arduous or ill-advised, we decline.

It is also satisfying to be wise enough to know that staying up very late or getting very drunk doesn't mean you had a good time, only that the following day is likely to be painful. Remember back when you realized that 'nothing good happens after 1am' and thought you were terribly mature for ducking out before the inevitably messy 3am conclusion? How amusing. It turns out that there are few things so enjoyable that they cannot be concluded by 11pm. Well, 10pm, ideally.

Another joy of getting older is feeling no pressure to impress when friends come round for a meal. That fashionable new cookbook with all the recipes made from hard-to-spell ingredients it would take most of Saturday to source? Look at the lovely pictures but do not attempt to create these dishes. They do not represent real life. Some women have known this all along, but for others, realizing that no one need ever make a souffle, filo pastry from scratch or individual themed place settings is something of a eureka moment. The supermarket sells prawn rings, most people like cheese and so long as there is something nice to drink, all will be well. Wise older women know: fun is so much better than perfect.

I've realized I need to seek
professional help. From a PA,
a chef and a housekeeper, ideally.

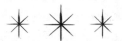

Home is where you don't
have to wear a bra.

Life has never given me lemons.
It has given me an ironic sense of
humour, bad posture and a short
temper, but literally no lemons.

'At every party there are two kinds of people – those who want to go home and those who don't. The trouble is, they are usually married to each other.'

Ann Landers

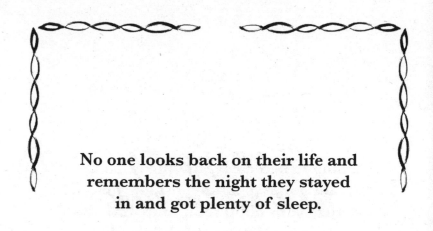

No one looks back on their life and
remembers the night they stayed
in and got plenty of sleep.

You're only as strong as the drinks
you pour, the tables you dance on
and the friends you party with.

There is no such thing
as an embarrassing situation,
only a great anecdote.

Going to bed early, staying at home, not going to a party: when you realize your childhood punishments have become your adult goals.

Better days are coming. They are called Saturday and Sunday.

Knowledge is like underwear: useful to have but not necessary to show off.

'What will you drink if you stop drinking?'

Patsy Stone, *Absolutely Fabulous*

'I think there are West End productions that are done with less preparation than Christmas. And less expense. And last a bit longer.'

Jenny Eclair

We eventually reach an age where we
go from 'I probably shouldn't say that'
to 'Well, let's see what happens ...'

If it involves fake smiling
then I'm not going.

I don't like the word 'lazy'. I call
it 'selective participation'.

Cinderella never asked for a prince.
She wanted a night off and a dress.

Common sense is like deodorant:
the people who need it most
never use it.

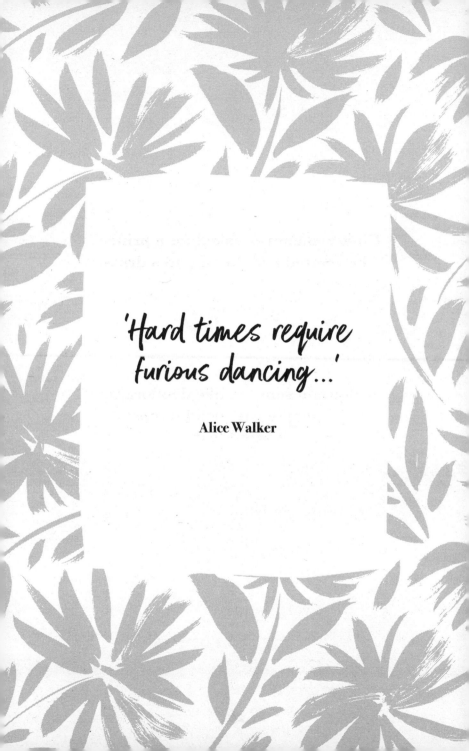

'Hard times require
furious dancing...'

Alice Walker

The art of the 'midlife crisis'

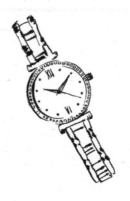

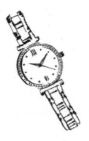

This terribly misnamed phenomenon is due a rebrand.
Firstly, it does not have to be undertaken in 'midlife'
— whenever that is — you may have one whenever you
wish. Also, 'crisis' should be replaced by 'opportunity'.

The term does not refer here to your friend's husband's
rather embarrassing flirtation with women in the
newsagents, nor his dalliance with unflattering denim, of
course. No. This is more of an 'everyday life sabbatical'.
It's about taking some time to embrace a part of your
personality that may have lain dormant and perhaps
taking up or revisiting an activity. To the surprise of some
and mild horror of your children, if possible. It is a way
of reminding others — and perhaps yourself, if necessary —
that getting older does not mean doing the same old, same
old from now until, well, the inevitable.

Maturity is not a synonym for boring and while we may have acres of common sense, that does not mean we must always be sensible.

Whether they take up an unusual hobby, decide to go backpacking for a year or buy a sports car, do not forget to support your friends in their own life sabbaticals, as it can be very enjoyable for all concerned. Who knows, you may receive an invitation to go stand-up paddleboarding, meet a friend in Kerala for a week or take a road trip. Of course, anything beyond the pale (e.g. military re-enactment, zorbing, swinging) will need to be politely declined, but as far as is reasonable, we should say yes to these adventures and expect our good friends to do the same for us. A rebranded 'later-life opportunity' is all sorts of fun.

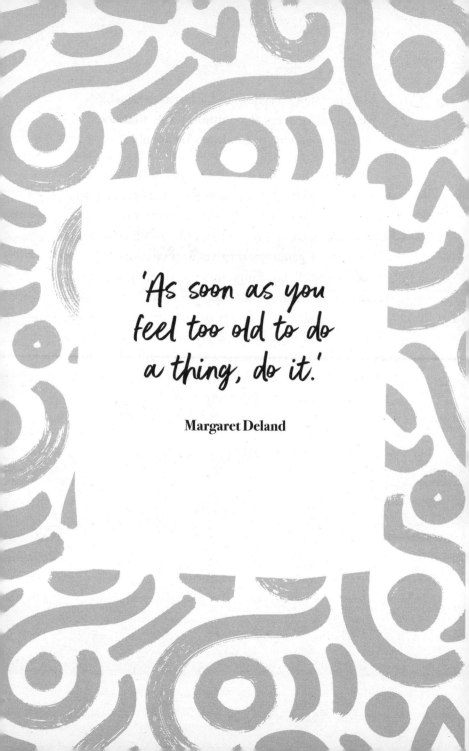

'As soon as you feel too old to do a thing, do it.'

Margaret Deland

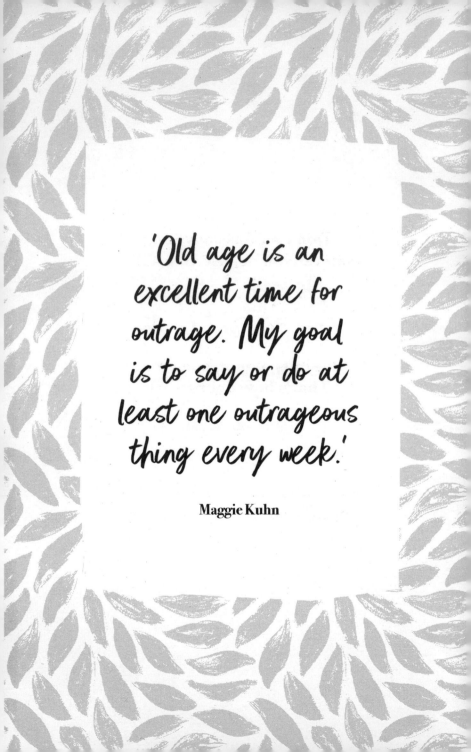

'Old age is an excellent time for outrage. My goal is to say or do at least one outrageous thing every week.'

Maggie Kuhn

Don't half-ass anything.
Whatever you do, use your full ass.

If life shuts a door, open it again.
That's how doors work.

We're all mature until someone
brings out the bubble wrap.

You don't necessarily become wiser with age. There are simply fewer stupid things left that you haven't already done.

Don't worry what people think: they mostly aren't.

'Some people are old when they're 18 and some people are young when they're 90. You can't define people by whatever society determines as their age. Time is a concept that human beings created.'

Yoko Ono

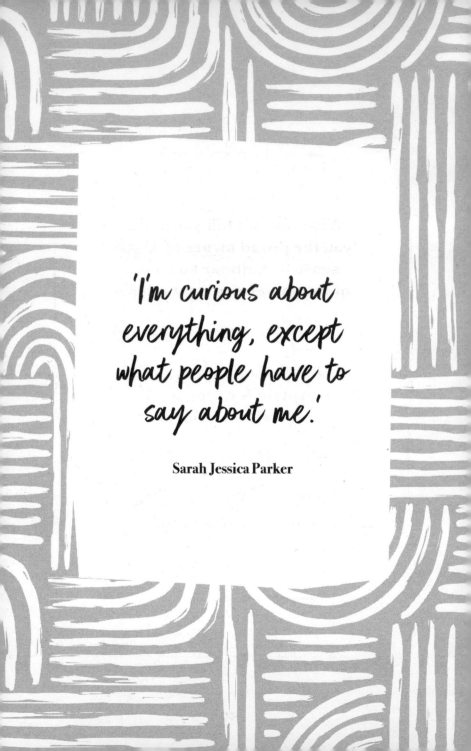

'I'm curious about everything, except what people have to say about me.'

Sarah Jessica Parker

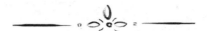

What doesn't kill you makes
you the proud owner of a dark
sense of humour and some
questionable coping methods.

I can explain it to you but I can't
understand it for you.

Life is a journey. Wear comfy shoes.

Sometimes I just have to tell myself:
it's not worth the jail time.

- - — - ✦ - ✦ - - ✦

Well-behaved women seldom
make history.

- - - — ✦ — - - ✦ - — - - —

There is nothing wrong with
talking to yourself. Sometimes
you need expert advice.

- - - — ✦ - — - -

'It's amazing what you can get if you quietly, clearly and authoritatively demand it.'

Meryl Streep

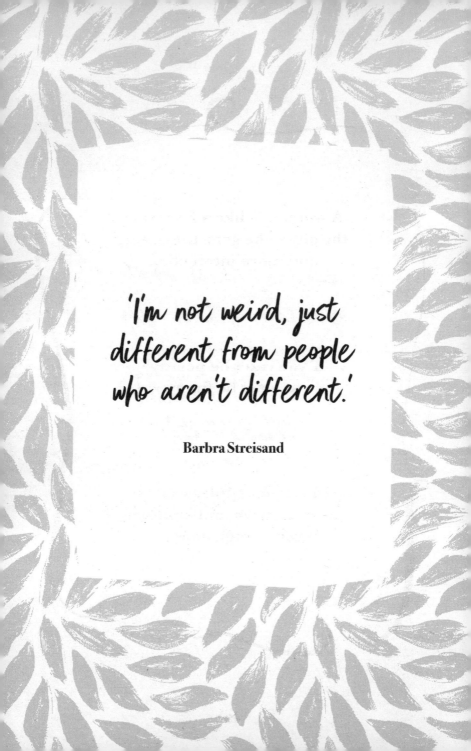

'I'm not weird, just different from people who aren't different.'

Barbra Streisand

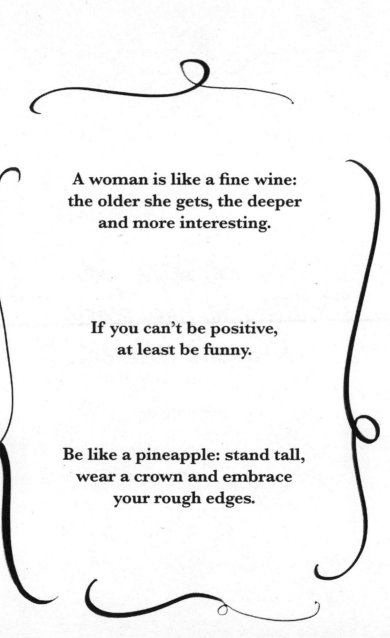

A woman is like a fine wine:
the older she gets, the deeper
and more interesting.

If you can't be positive,
at least be funny.

Be like a pineapple: stand tall,
wear a crown and embrace
your rough edges.

Technology

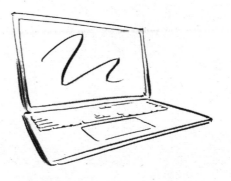

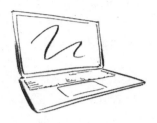

Helpless technophobes. Left behind by the fast-moving
modern world. Intimidated by any task that can only
be carried out via the internet. All are enduring cliches
about the older woman, and very useful they are too.
We can of course figure it out if we have to – we have
tackled far bigger challenges in our time. But the truth is
that we simply don't want to. It is often very boring and,
after all, that is what young people are for. Fortunately,
they usually fail to notice that we are more than capable
of wrangling technology when it suits us, such as
searching Netflix for the new series featuring that very
attractive actor, ordering a takeaway and not leaving the
wine off the online shop.

'Grandma, why don't you just download the app?'
'Mum, you just have to set up an online
account and it will be so much easier.'

Will it, dear? That sounds wonderful. What would be *even* easier is if you would just do it for me. Let me just assume my confused and helpless face and I'll go do something more interesting while you take care of it. If you annoy me further in this matter then I shall be sure to comment on your every Instagram post and embarrass you horribly. I'm afraid I *do* know how to do that.

As older women, we possess a skill set younger generations can only dream of. We are comfortable talking to strangers on the phone, we know how to use a map that doesn't feature a blue dot marking our location and we don't spontaneously combust if the Wi-Fi is down. And for everything else, we have young people. It's the perfect set-up. Once you have reached a certain age, you have earned the right never to have to do anything as tedious as set up a new iPhone.

If you are ever caught using technology in a way you had implied was far beyond you, threatening to blow your cover, then a good tactic is to immediately hold your phone above your head and walk slowly around the room, claiming you are trying to 'charge' the signal.* The eye-rolling from your nearest and dearest will confirm you are out of the woods and no one suspects a thing.

(*If you really want to confuse them, do it with the landline.)

'As a teenager you are at the last stage in your life when you will be happy to hear that the phone is for you.'

Fran Lebowitz

'I don't have pet peeves like some people. I have whole kennels of irritation.'

Whoopi Goldberg

Do anything well and you risk
someone asking you to do it again.

Some days I amaze myself. Other
days I find my keys in the fridge.

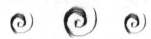

Some people just can't laugh at
themselves. That's where I come in.

Revenge is beneath me.
But accidents do happen.

Breathe in for five. Breathe out for
five. Now screw the deep breathing
and have a glass of wine.

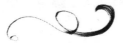

To confuse a child, simply tell them
you are older than the internet.

'For a list of all the ways technology has failed to improve the quality of life, please press three.'

Alice Kahn

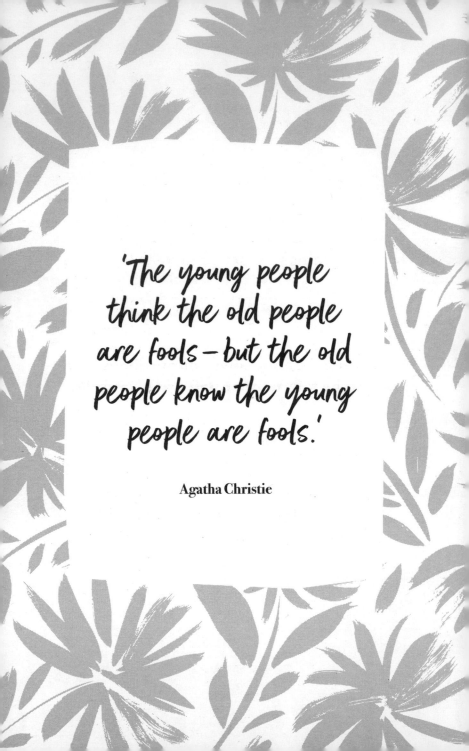

'The young people
think the old people
are fools – but the old
people know the young
people are fools.'

Agatha Christie

It's useful to organize tasks into categories: things I won't do now, things I won't do later and things I'll get someone else to do.

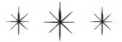

Alcohol will not solve your problems. But, to be fair, neither will water or milk.

I may not have lost all my marbles yet but there's a chance there is a hole in the bag somewhere.

The biggest lie we tell ourselves is,
'I don't need to write that
down, I'll remember.'

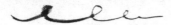

If you stare at something you dropped
on the floor for long enough, eventually
someone will pick it up for you.

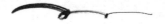

Don't make the same mistake twice. Make
it six or seven times just to be sure.

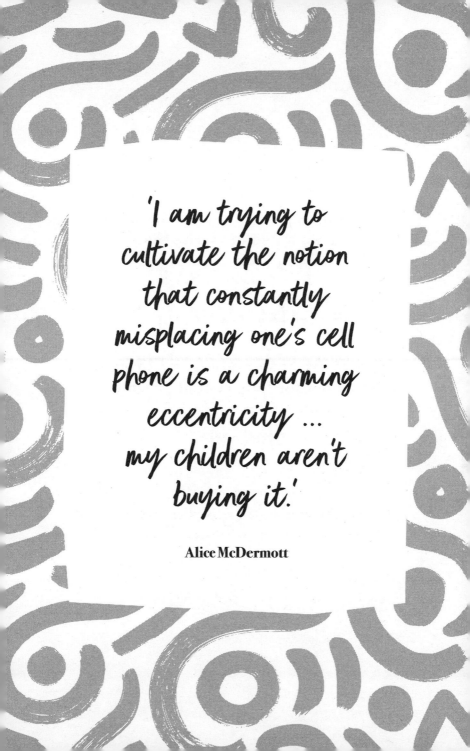

'I am trying to cultivate the notion that constantly misplacing one's cell phone is a charming eccentricity ... my children aren't buying it.'

Alice McDermott

'If television's a babysitter, the internet is a drunk librarian who won't shut up.'

Dorothy Gambrell

There is a difference between giving
up, knowing you've had enough
and not caring either way.

When something goes wrong in life,
sometimes you just have to shout,
'PLOT TWIST!' and move on.

I have neither the time nor the
crayons to explain this to you.

Friends

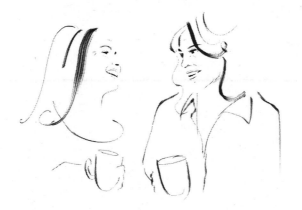

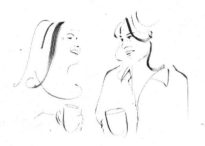

'For what do we live, but to make sport for our
neighbours, and laugh at them in our turn?' asked
Jane Austen's Mr Bennett in *Pride and Prejudice*.
Which seems a sensible way of looking at the world.
After all, getting older means accepting ourselves
and our friends for the glorious eccentrics we have
become. Now all the hypersensitivity of our younger
years is behind us, we can laugh at ourselves and
each other without anyone getting offended.

Our later years often mark the return of old friends
who have been away fighting in the trenches of
parenthood. It's not that we didn't see them in those
years that they, or we, or both of us, were bringing
up children, but there is only so much attention you
can give to even a very good friend while also trying

to stop a child putting small objects in their mouth/
electrocuting themselves/terrorizing the cat.

And of course we can and should continue to
make new friends. Our bullshit sensors are so well
tuned by years of experience that it becomes easy
to spot potential allies and partners in crime and
swerve those probably not on our wavelength.

When you are experienced enough to have stopped
bothering with anyone who is emotionally draining and
not a good friend, it frees up time to spend with those
wonderful people we love and very much like. (Or who
have been there from the beginning and we must keep
close as they know where all the bodies are buried.)

'Friendship is a wildly underrated medication.'

Anna Deavere Smith

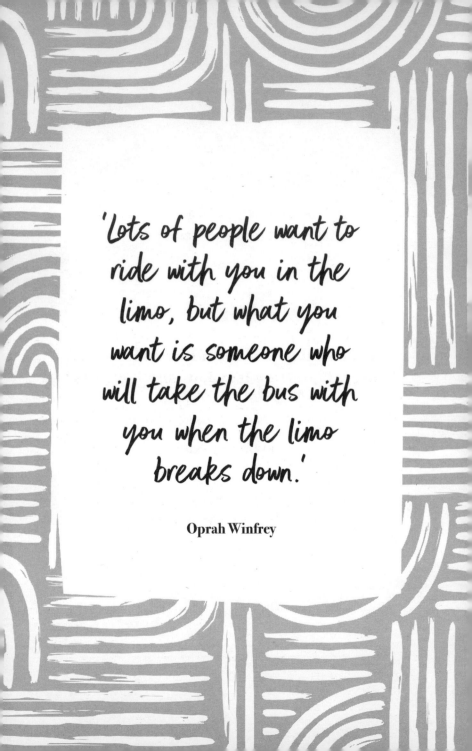

'Lots of people want to ride with you in the limo, but what you want is someone who will take the bus with you when the limo breaks down.'

Oprah Winfrey

True friends don't judge each other.
They judge others together.

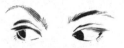

The glass may be half full or half empty.
The real question is: what is in the glass?

I'm sorry I got angry and said a
load of stuff I meant but probably
should have kept to myself.

Askhole: a person who
is constantly asking your advice
and never following it.

It's OK if someone doesn't like you.
Many people have terrible taste.

Friends are the people who stick by you
when you are right because anyone will
stick by you when you are wrong.

'The friend who holds your hand and says the wrong thing is made of dearer stuff than the one who stays away.'

Barbara Kingsolver

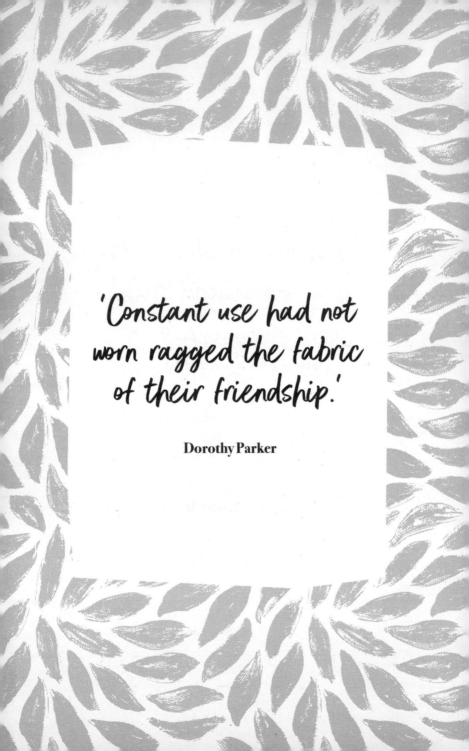

'Constant use had not worn ragged the fabric of their friendship.'

Dorothy Parker

Do no harm. Take no shit.

**Sorry I'm late. I got here as
soon as I wanted to.**

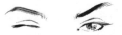

**I'm making some changes in my life.
So if you don't hear from me,
you're one of them.**

Age like wine, not like milk.

Good friends don't let you do
stupid things ... alone.

If you are required to go through hell, at
least walk in like you own the place.

'You find out who your real friends are when you're involved in a scandal.'

Elizabeth Taylor

'The best time to
make friends is before
you need them.'

Ethel Barrymore

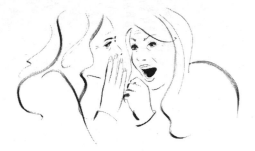

143 per cent of people exaggerate.

This 'killing them with kindness'
is taking way longer than
I had expected.

A friend is someone who bails you
out of jail. A best friend is the one
sitting beside you, shaking her
head, saying: 'Wow, crazy night!'

Appearance

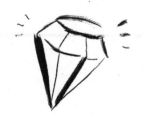

'God grant me the serenity to accept the things I cannot change, courage to change the things I can, and the wisdom to ignore those adverts for face cream that will make absolutely no difference whatsoever,' goes the older, wiser, fiercer woman's prayer.

One amusing lesson we learn with the advantage of age is that there really is nothing new. The first time a fashion from our youth comes back around and we spot teenagers in something we wore twenty years ago, it feels rather unsettling. Particularly if they have the temerity to label it 'vintage'. By the third time, however, having an original of a now-coveted item lurking in the back of our wardrobe makes us feel cool, and knowing we have the good sense not to wear something so impractical/uncomfortable again makes us feel smug.

None of us are above a little vanity now and again. And we can hardly be blamed for occasionally falling for some marketing spiel, promising to make something firmer/tauter/brighter. But really, the most effective 'anti-ageing' treatment is not giving a hoot. Yes, there are times we glimpse our reflection in a shop window and wonder who that older lady is, but serums, creams and expensive treatments be damned. All we need is a sense of humour, the right attitude … and, OK, a good pair of tweezers. Plus, it's much harder to ironically raise an eyebrow after having Botox.

'If your hair is done
and you're wearing
good shoes, you
can get away with
anything.'

Iris Apfel

'People are always asking me, "What do you want people to say about you a hundred years from now?" I always say I want them to say, "Dang, don't she still look good for her age?"

Dolly Parton

A diamond is just a lump of coal that
performed well under pressure.

I don't even believe myself when
I say I'll be ready in five minutes.

Raise your hand if you have an opinion
about me. Now put it over your mouth.

The best things in life are actually often quite expensive.

I'm 90 per cent sunshine and 10 per cent hurricane.

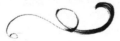

I'm still hot (it just comes in flashes now).

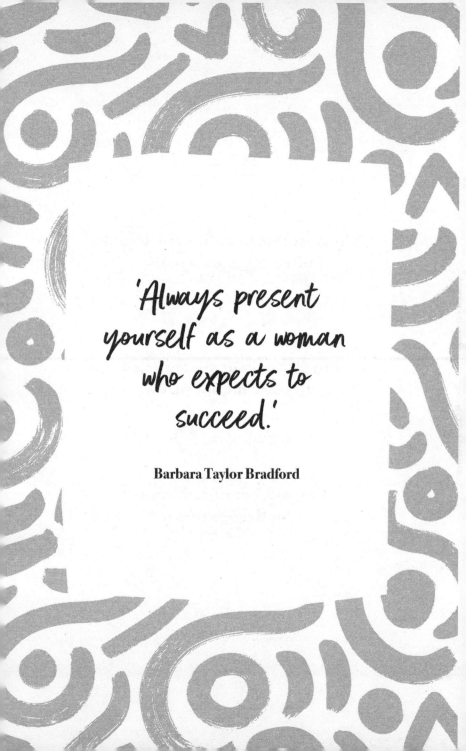

'Always present yourself as a woman who expects to succeed.'

Barbara Taylor Bradford

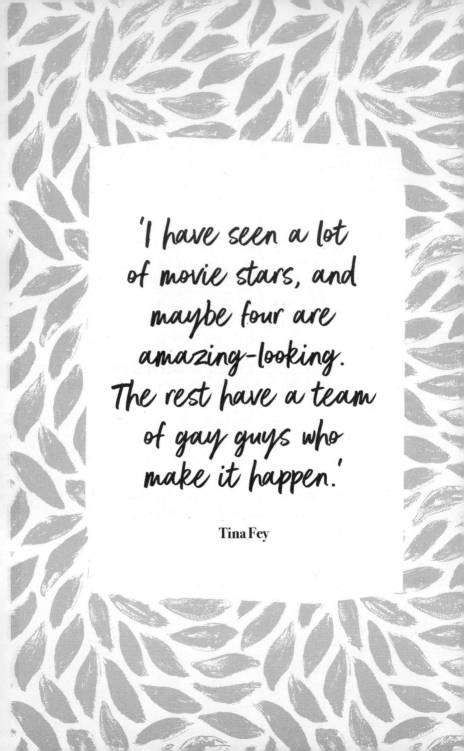

'I have seen a lot
of movie stars, and
maybe four are
amazing-looking.
The rest have a team
of gay guys who
make it happen.'

Tina Fey

The older you get, the better
you get. Unless you are a banana.

My dentist told me I needed a crown.
Finally, someone realized.

Sometimes you're the windshield;
sometimes you're the bug.

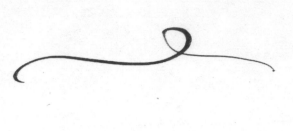

Dance like no one is watching.
Sing like no one can hear you.
Walk like your tights aren't
falling down.

'Awesome' ends in 'me'.
Coincidence? I think not.

Seize the day. Don't be one
of the women who turned down
dessert on the *Titanic*.

'It is best to act with confidence, no matter how little right you have to it.'

Lillian Hellman

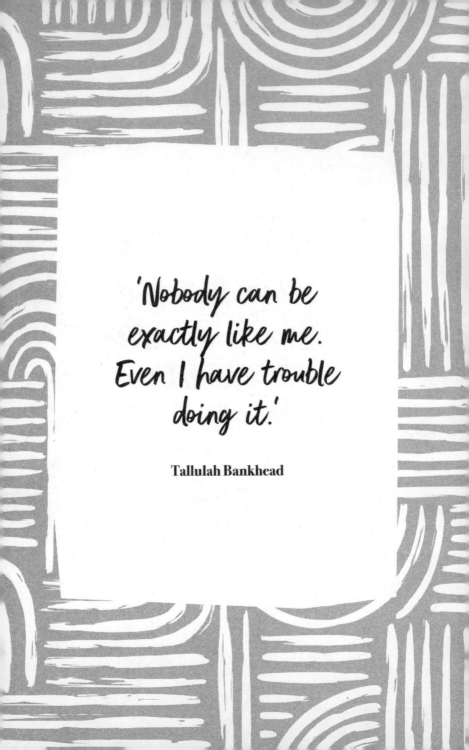

'Nobody can be
exactly like me.
Even I have trouble
doing it.'

Tallulah Bankhead

Avoid negative people, dull situations
and overhead fluorescent lighting.

I don't have grey hair; I have
wisdom highlights.

Young at heart and only slightly
older in other places.

Health and fitness

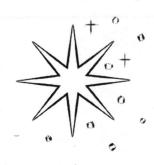

It can feel like there are some irritating barriers to entry as an older woman when it comes to exercise. Gym kit often seems designed exclusively for the young and lithe, in colours so bright they can be seen from space. There are now apparently 378 different types of yoga you must choose from and, bafflingly, something called a 'juice cleanse'. And no one wants to be patronized at the gym by a young man with absurdly overdeveloped arm muscles (unless he is very, *very* attractive).

But even in the arena of health and fitness – apparently now called 'wellbeing' – which seems so set up for the young, age and wisdom is an advantage. For one, when you have lived through every fad from the cabbage soup diet to Atkins, you have a highly developed ability to recognize absolute nonsense when you see it. No, that diet is not going to give you 'defined abs in three weeks'; it will make you miserable and give you terrible wind.

We also have realistic expectations and know that the secret to staying active is to find something you like to do and stick to it. Of course, if you enjoy a 6am spin class then more power to you. For the rest of us, it is very liberating to ditch all pretence that we are going to get up early and go for a jog and instead go for walk with our friends, play a sport we like or dance around the kitchen while we cook, embarrassing any children or grandchildren in the vicinity to the best of our abilities.

'Don't waste so much time thinking about how much you weigh. There is no more mind-numbing, boring, idiotic, self-destructive diversion from the fun of living.'

Meryl Streep

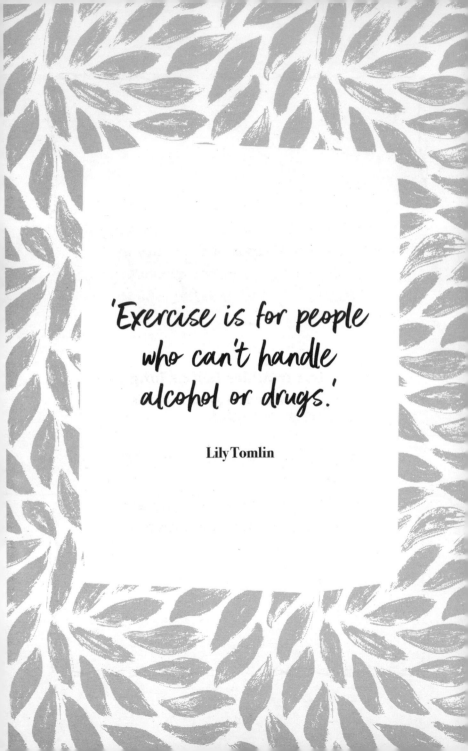

'Exercise is for people
who can't handle
alcohol or drugs.'

Lily Tomlin

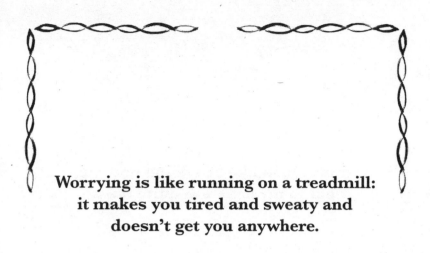

Worrying is like running on a treadmill:
it makes you tired and sweaty and
doesn't get you anywhere.

May your troubles last as long as
your New Year's resolutions.

If you don't like where you are,
move. You are not a tree.

It may look like I'm doing nothing,
but in my head I'm quite busy.

Know which dreams are worth
pursuing: there is no pot of gold at the
end of the rainbow but there may be a
cookie in the back of the cupboard.

I get most of my exercise these days
through shaking my head in disbelief.

'We are always the same age inside.'

Gertrude Stein

'The only way I'll ever run a marathon is if I'm involved in the administration.'

Sally Phillips

Not waving, not drowning, just
trying to get rid of this wasp.

Strength is the ability to break a chocolate
bar into four pieces with your bare hands
and then just eat one of those pieces.

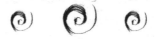

I don't let my age define me,
but the side-effects are getting
harder to ignore.

To be old and wise, first you have to be young and stupid.

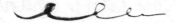

You may call it 'revenge'; I call it 'returning the favour'.

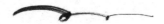

Exercise? Oh sorry, I thought you said *accessorize*.

'If you can't change
your fate, change
your attitude.'

Amy Tan

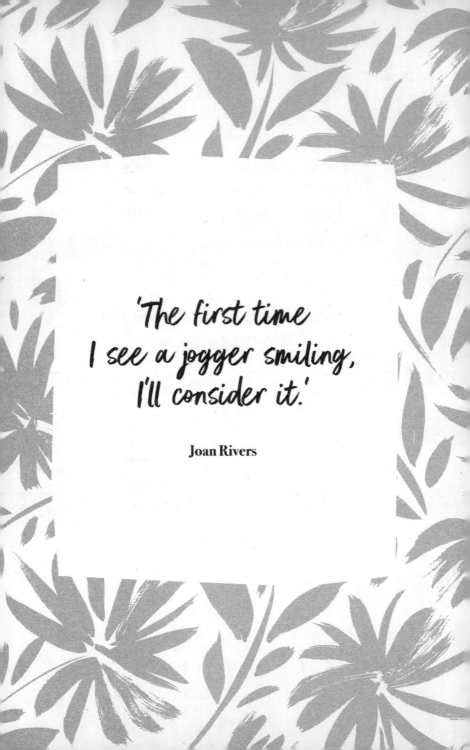

'The first time
I see a jogger smiling,
I'll consider it.'

Joan Rivers

I'm in a really good place right
now. I don't mean emotionally,
I mean I'm in the wine store.

— - — — — — - —

It's better to slow down
than break down.

— - — — — — - — — — — — — — —

If you were able to believe in Santa
Claus for eight years, you can believe
in yourself for five minutes.

— - — — — — - —

Dating

Being single can be a delight at any age. There's the freedom to do what you want, watch what you want with a plate of whatever you like on your lap, with the only key disadvantages if you live alone being it's always your turn to take the bin out and there's no one to call your phone if you can't find it. The world of dating, however, can be very trying, no matter how old you are.

Some people will argue that young people have ruined dating with their apps, stripping away all nuance and spontaneity. Others are of the opinion that chatting to a possible suitor online, establishing that they are probably not a lunatic/bore/serial killer before spending valuable time meeting them is both efficient and preferable to many alternatives, such as hanging around in a bar to be chatted up by an account manager with halitosis.

But whatever your views, if you are navigating the weird world of dating, at least you are doing it as a wise older woman, in possession of a high level of experience and a low tolerance for nonsense. Rather than thinking, 'They would like me if I were thinner/smarter/more expensively dressed,' we now realize that, 'They would like me if they had better taste.' That's not say we don't still make mistakes – deliberate or otherwise – but you have the confidence to know when it's not you, it's most definitely them.

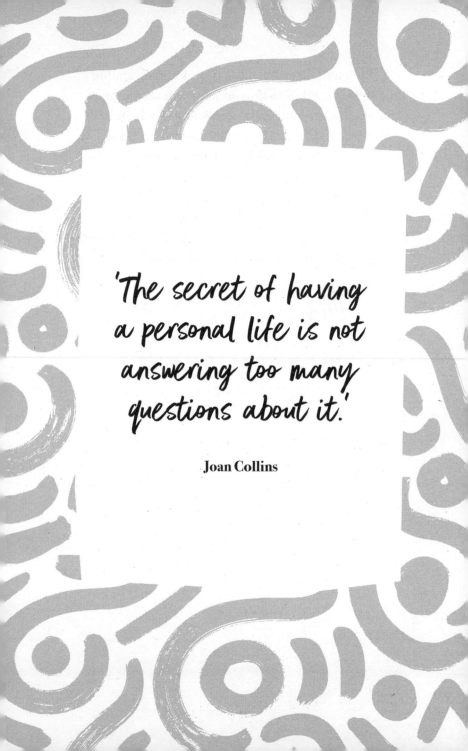

'The secret of having
a personal life is not
answering too many
questions about it.'

Joan Collins

'My philosophy for dating is just to fart right away.'

Jenny McCarthy

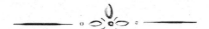

Everyone was thinking it;
I just said it.

I am always on the lookout
for fools not to suffer.

When dating, a man wearing
a ring is to be avoided. Either he's
married or he's the kind of man
who likes to wear rings.

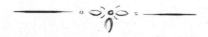

Life is not a fairy tale. If you lose your shoe at midnight you are drunk.

—————————

Some people are like clouds. They disappear and it's a beautiful day.

—————————

There are over 7 trillion nerves in the human body and some people manage to get on every single one.

'I never trusted good-
looking boys.'

Frances McDormand

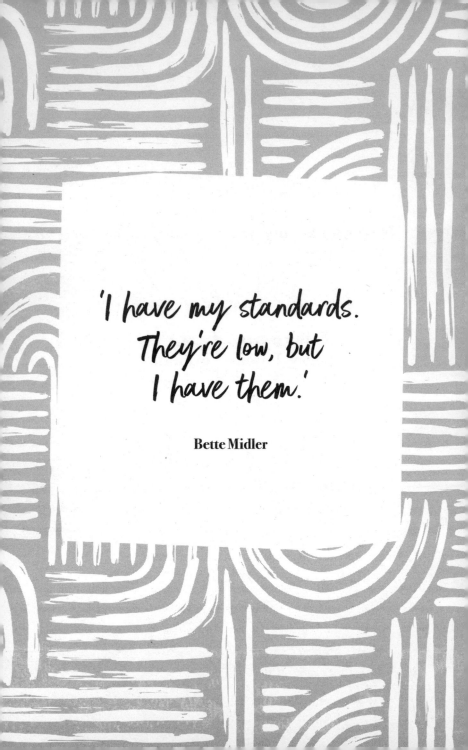

'I have my standards.
They're low, but
I have them.'

Bette Midler

Never let anyone waste your time twice.

**Failure is not an option.
Sorry, I meant 'optional'.**

**I forgive myself for not being
perfect. But that doesn't mean I
have to forgive anyone else.**

Everyone has the capacity to bring happiness. Some when they arrive, others when they leave.

My mistakes don't define me. My jokes do.

Please cancel my subscriptions to your issues.

'Love affairs are the real only education in life.'

Marlene Dietrich

'Far too many people are looking for the right person, instead of trying to be the right person.'

Gloria Steinem

If two wrongs don't make a right,
try three.

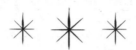

I pity the person who fails to see
what a funny, clever badass I am.

Why is it that when you finally get to
the point where you can do anything
you want, you are too tired to do it?

Relationships

There is a reason why romcoms always end
with the couple getting together – because
it's mostly hard work from there on in.

For many of us, though, relationships do get easier
with age, whether we have been together for a long
time or a short time. Remember when you were
young and you would dump someone for wearing
embarrassing shoes, not having heard of your favourite
band or pronouncing 'particularly' incorrectly? Oh,
what small misdemeanours these seem now, as we sit
and watch the hair grow from our loved one's ears!

Now our expectations are more realistic. We know
what is important to us in life in general, and this
includes relationships. We know what to bring up
and let go. And also what we can reasonably expect

from the person who we put down as our next of kin on all the forms. Yes, they need to pull their weight around the house. But equally, if their face is a picture of horror when we mention a trip to the antiques market, we probably don't mind if they stay home.

Whether we have been with the same person for years and weathered storms together (and probably some frosty periods, and plenty of mildly overcast days) or we have just got together with someone new, we have our standards while understanding that people have their off days and no one is perfect. Even, we grudgingly admit, us.

'I love being married.
It's so great to find
one special person you
want to annoy for the
rest of your life.'

Rita Rudner

'Honesty is the key to
a great relationship.
If you can fake that,
you're in!'

Courtney Cox

You don't have to attend every
argument you are invited to.

A husband is a person who helps a woman
overcome difficulties that never would
have arisen if he were not her husband.

Failure is like manure. Sure, it stinks,
but things grow as a result.

It's better to ask for forgiveness
than permission.

Silence is golden. Alternatively,
duct tape is silver.

The definition of false hope:
putting items on the stairs for your
family members to carry up.

'My heart's in the right place. I know, 'cuz I hid it there.'

Carrie Fisher

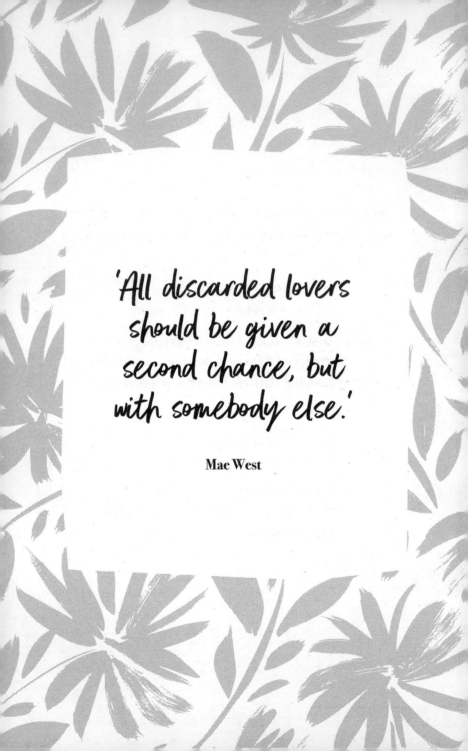

'All discarded lovers
should be given a
second chance, but
with somebody else.'

Mae West

My style of housework is best described
as, 'There seems to have been a struggle'.

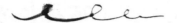

If you watch *Die Hard* straight after
Love Actually, Alan Rickman is punished
for what he did to Emma Thompson.

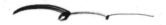

Life will always throw things at
you. Learn to duck quickly and
they will hit someone else.

If anyone ever asks who your favourite child is, try to pick one of your own.

I don't like morning people.
Or mornings. Or people.

In December, shout, 'Don't come in here!' and everyone will assume you are wrapping presents rather than drinking wine and watching *Bridgerton* in peace.

'The trouble with some women is that they get all excited about nothing—and then marry him.'

Cher

'Relationship gurus always said that an attraction based on friendship and mutual respect was far more likely to stay the course—and the bastards were right.'

Marian Keyes

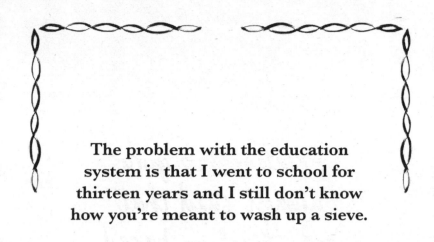

The problem with the education
system is that I went to school for
thirteen years and I still don't know
how you're meant to wash up a sieve.

When tempted to fight fire with
fire, remember that the Fire
Service usually uses water.

I am wholly uncompetitive.
Unless there is a chance
I might win.

Grandparenting

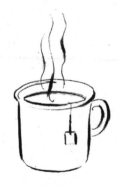

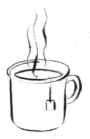

To grandparent: verb. To provide free childcare, support and advice (largely ignored) to your child or similar close younger person in your life in the event of them becoming a parent.

When our children become parents themselves, we hope that this will give them a fresh insight into all the hard work, sacrifice and unselfish love we poured into their childhoods. Realistically, it's more likely that they ignore the fact that we have been there, done that, and patronize the hell out of us. They don't want to hear about how parenting was done in our day, appearing to view it as borderline cruelty and a health and safety nightmare. But we forgive them, as we remember what it was like to be the sleep-deprived parent of a young child. (Well, mostly. Some of it we had to forget for the sake of our sanity.)

Grandchildren are a wonderful gift in so many ways. You get to enjoy their energy, their curiosity and the mad things they say, then hand them back to their parents. You can ignore their nap times and let them do things their mum and dad don't. However, it's also true that they can be exhausting, badly behaved and remind you how glad you are that your parenting days are behind you. If you do have young children in your life then embrace being their cool, fun, bad-ass gran. If you don't, embrace the fact that you can own a cream sofa, don't get asked to babysit last minute when you already have plans and never feel obliged to stick terrible finger paintings on your fridge.

'Look, you didn't ask me for my opinion, but I'm old, so I'm giving it anyway.'

Sophia, *Golden Girls*

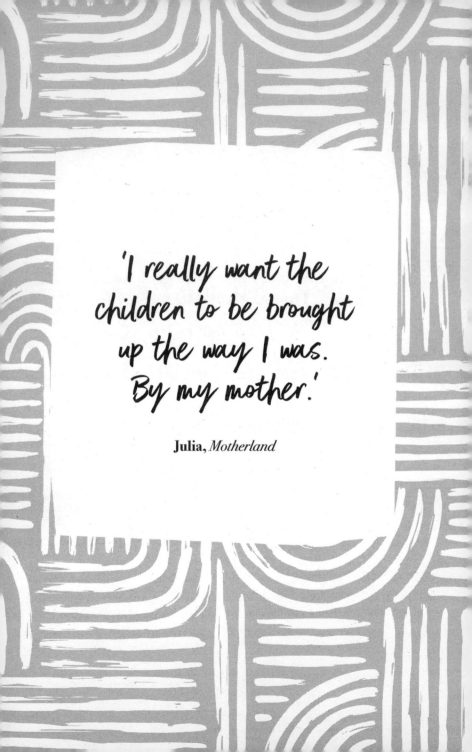

'I really want the children to be brought up the way I was. By my mother.'

Julia, *Motherland*

Act like you know what you are
doing. Then people will think you
know what you are doing.

Why do people say,
'Go big or go home'? Home, please.
That's been my goal all day.

When making a decision, I vow
to never forget to ask the most
important question: will it be fun?

Most people seem normal until
you get to know them.

Do you remember when you were
a kid and everyone praised you
when you took a long nap?

'Becoming a grandmother is wonderful. One moment you're just a mother. The next you are all-wise and prehistoric.'

Pam Brown

'A grandparent is old on the outside but young on the inside. If your baby is "beautiful and perfect, never cries or fusses, sleeps on schedule and burps on demand, an angel all the time", you're the grandma.'

Teresa Bloomingdale

Ageing is inevitable.
Getting old is a choice.

— - — - — - — - —

I'm doing an escape room today.
Well, actually it's work but I'm
pretty sure I can get out of it.

— - — - — - — - — - — - —

Tact means the ability to tell someone
to go to hell in such a way that they
look forward to the journey.

— - — - — - — -

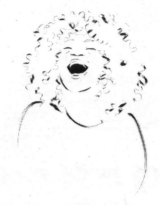

The wine made me do it.

'Every house needs a
grandmother in it.'

Louisa May Alcott

'When I see my parents letting my kids eat their body weight in ice cream, telling them they don't have to bother with homework, I think, "Who are these people and where were they when I was growing up?"'

Sindhu Vee

**Whatever hits the fan will not
be distributed evenly.**

**A meeting without snacks
should be an email.**

**It's important not to let things
get you down. Not when it's
this hard to get back up.**

Never underestimate
the potential for stupidity
of people in large groups.

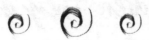

I may be a natural empath, but
I can still choose not to give a shit.

'I love children,
the only problem with
children: they grow
up to be people.'

Betty White

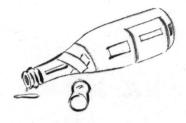

**Let's drink champagne
and dance on tables.**